JUICES FOR RENAL

HEALTH

Managing chronic kidney disease

with natural juices

Dr Kelly Hart

TABLE OF CONTENTSs

CHAPTER 1

The kidney and its function

The kidneys are two bean-shaped organs located on either side of the spine in the abdominal cavity. They are responsible for filtering waste products and extra fluid from the blood and disposing of them in the form of urine.

The kidneys also produce several hormones that regulate blood pressure, red blood cell production, and calcium metabolism. The kidneys are made up of millions of tiny filtering units called nephrons.

Each nephron consists of a tuft of capillaries (glomerulus) surrounded by a cup-like structure (Bowman's capsule). Blood enters the glomerulus and is filtered into the Bowman's capsule, with waste products and extra fluid entering the urine.

The urine passes down a tube called the ureter to the bladder, where it is stored until it is released from the body. The main functions of the kidneys include: Filtering waste products and extra fluid from the blood: The kidneys filter out toxins, waste products, and extra fluid from the blood and release them in the form of urine. Regulating blood pressure: They produce a hormone called renin, which helps regulate blood pressure. Renin causes the blood vessels to constrict, resulting in an increase in blood pressure.

The kidneys also produce a hormone called calcitriol, which helps regulate calcium and phosphorus levels in the blood. Maintaining electrolyte balance:

Regulating the levels of electrolytes such as sodium, potassium, and chloride in the body is also a function of the kidneys

The kidneys are essential for the body to function properly. Damage to the kidneys can result in a number of serious health problems, including high blood pressure, anemia, and electrolyte imbalances.

Therefore, it is important to take care of your kidneys and keep them healthy. Eating a healthy diet, exercising regularly, and avoiding smoking and excessive alcohol consumption can help keep your kidneys healthy.

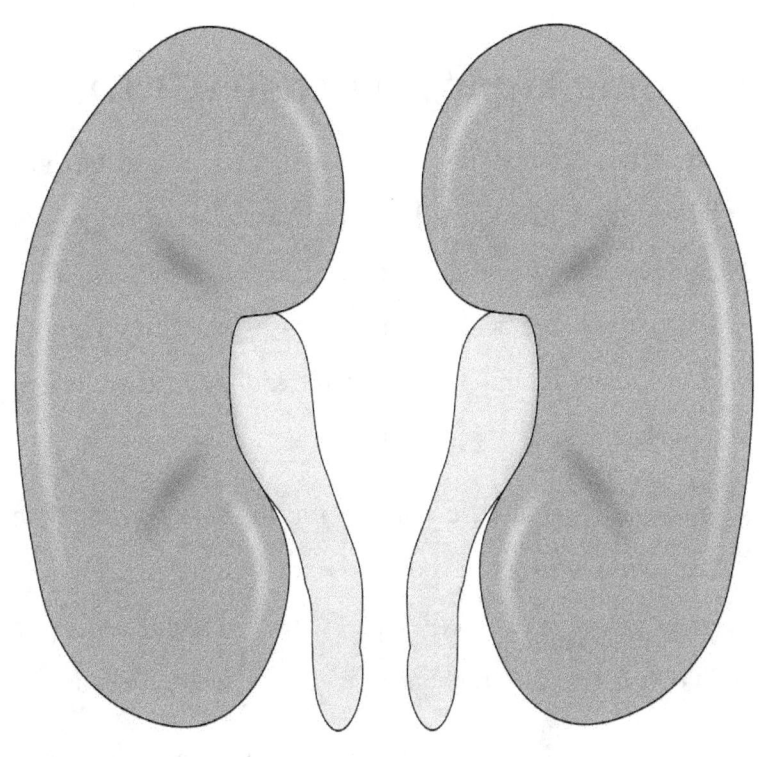

CHAPTER 2

Chronic kidney disease (CKD)

Kidney disease, also known as renal disease, is a medical condition in which the kidneys fail to adequately filter out waste products from the blood. The two main types of kidney disease are acute kidney disease, which is an abrupt loss of kidney function, and chronic kidney disease, which is a long-term loss of kidney function.

Chronic kidney disease can be further divided into five stages, with stage five being the most severe. Common causes of acute and chronic kidney disease include diabetes, high blood pressure, infections, and drug or toxin exposure.

Other causes of kidney disease include genetic disorders, autoimmune diseases, and blockages in the urinary tract. While kidney disease can be treated with medications and lifestyle changes, some of these conditions may progress to end-stage renal disease, requiring dialysis or a kidney transplant. For patients with chronic kidney disease, lifestyle changes such as following a low-sodium diet, quitting smoking, and exercising regularly can help to slow the progression of the disease.

Medications, such as ACE inhibitors and angiotensin receptor blockers, can help to control blood pressure, while diuretics can help to reduce excess fluid in the body.

In severe cases, dialysis may be necessary to filter waste products from the blood. In end-stage renal disease, a kidney transplant may be the only option for survival.

We are going to discuss about the chronic kidney disease and possible ways to curb it naturally using homemade fruits and vegetables juices.

CHAPTER 3

Stages of chronic kidney diseases

The five stages of chronic kidney disease (CKD) are a progressive decline in kidney function that occurs over time. The stages are classified by the glomerular filtration rate (GFR), which measures how well the kidneys remove waste and excess fluid from the body.

Stage 1 (GFR 90+)

In this stage, the Stage 1 (GFR 90+) of chronic kidney disease is characterized by a decrease in the glomerular filtration rate (GFR) below 90 milliliters per minute (ml/min).

At this stage, the kidneys are still functioning properly and there is little to no damage to the kidneys. In this stage, the kidneys are still able to filter and remove waste and excess fluid from the blood, but at a reduced rate. This can cause an increase in the levels of certain substances, such as creatinine, in the blood. Other symptoms may include swelling (edema), increased blood pressure, fatigue, and poor appetite.

Treatment at this stage is focused on controlling and managing the symptoms, slowing down the progression of the disease, and preventing further damage to the kidneys. This includes lifestyle modifications such as reducing salt intake, maintaining a healthy weight, and controlling blood pressure, as well as medications to control blood pressure and cholesterol levels.

Regular monitoring of kidney function is also important to ensure the disease does not progress to more advanced stages.

Stage 2 (GFR 60-89)

Stage 2 of chronic kidney disease (CKD) is characterized by a glomerular filtration rate (GFR) between 60 and 89. This stage is considered mild to moderate kidney damage, and is usually diagnosed through tests like a urine albumin-to-creatinine ratio or a serum creatinine test.

In this stage, the kidneys are still able to filter out wastes and extra fluid, but they are not functioning optimally. People with Stage 2 CKD should take steps to improve their kidney health by eating a healthy diet that is low in sodium, fat, and cholesterol; getting regular exercise; and maintaining a healthy weight.

It is also important to talk to a doctor about any medications that may be contributing to the progression of kidney disease.

There may be alternative treatments or medications that can help. In this stage, it is important to monitor kidney function closely and to pay attention to any symptoms of kidney damage. These can include increased fatigue, decreased appetite, swelling in the legs and ankles, and increased protein in the urine.

If the condition worsens, the patient may need to begin dialysis or consider a kidney transplant. By taking preventive measures and managing the disease, people with Stage 2 CKD can often slow or even stop the progression of kidney damage.

Early interventions can make a huge difference in how the kidneys function in the future and in the patient's overall health.

Stage 3 (GFR 30-59)

Stage 3 of chronic kidney disease (CKD) is defined as having a Glomerular Filtration Rate (GFR) of 30-59. This stage is considered to be mild to moderate kidney damage and is often termed "moderate CKD."

During this stage, the kidneys are still able to adequately filter out waste and fluids from the body, but the damage is beginning to become more severe. Symptoms of stage 3 CKD may include fatigue, a decrease in appetite, swelling in the hands and feet, muscle cramps, difficulty sleeping, anemia, and nausea.

In this stage, it is important to make lifestyle changes to slow the progression of the disease. This includes eating a healthy, balanced diet, avoiding processed foods, limiting sodium and phosphorus intake, and reducing alcohol consumption.

Exercise is also beneficial in helping to reduce symptoms and improve overall health. It is important to have regular check-ups with your doctor to make sure your kidney function is staying stable.

Overall, stage 3 CKD is a serious condition that requires proper management in order to prevent further damage to the kidneys. It is important to make lifestyle changes to ensure that the kidneys are functioning normally.

Stage 4 (GFR 15-29)

Stage 4 of chronic kidney disease is a serious health condition in which the kidneys' ability to filter waste from the body is significantly reduced.

At this stage, the glomerular filtration rate (GFR) is between 15 and 29. In this stage, the kidneys are unable to handle the waste and fluids which can lead to an accumulation of toxins in the body.

This can cause a range of health issues, such as high blood pressure, anemia, and bone and mineral disorders. It also increases the risk of developing cardiovascular disease, stroke, and kidney failure.

It is important for someone with stage 4 chronic kidney disease to work with a medical team to find the best treatment plan. This may include a combination of lifestyle changes, medications, and potentially dialysis or a kidney transplant.

Lifestyle changes may include eating a healthy diet, getting regular exercise, and managing stress. Medications can help to manage symptoms, slow the progression of the disease, and reduce the risk of complications.

Dialysis or a transplant may be needed if the disease has progressed to a point where the kidneys are no longer able to adequately filter the body's waste.

It is also important for someone with stage 4 chronic kidney disease to attend regular checkups and follow their doctor's advice. This will help to monitor the progression of the disease and ensure that any necessary treatments are started in time.

With proper medical care, lifestyle changes, and medications, someone with stage 4 chronic kidney disease can often manage the condition and improve their quality of life.

Stage 5 (GFR <15)

End-stage renal disease (ESRD) is the most serious form of CKD and requires dialysis or a kidney transplant to maintain life. CKD develops slowly and can be managed through diet, lifestyle changes, and medications.

Early detection and treatment can help slow the progression of the disease and improve quality of life. Stage 5 of Chronic Kidney Disease (CKD) is the most serious stage of kidney disease.

At this stage, the GFR (glomerular filtration rate) is below 15, meaning that the kidneys are no longer able to adequately filter out wastes and other toxins from the body. This can lead to a buildup of toxins in the body, as well as an increased risk for other health complications.

Common symptoms of Stage 5 CKD include fatigue, loss of appetite, nausea, difficulty sleeping, and swelling in the extremities. Other complications can include high blood pressure, anemia, and proteinuria. At this stage, the only viable treatment option is dialysis or a kidney transplant. Dialysis is a process of filtering and removing toxins from the blood, while a kidney transplant is a surgical procedure to replace the diseased kidney with a healthy one.

Both of these treatments are expensive and time-consuming, and require a lifelong commitment to managing treatment and monitoring health.

Regular visits to the doctor are also essential in order to monitor organ function and to adjust medication dosages as needed.

CHAPTER 4

Juices for kidney health

Juices can be an effective way to help manage kidney diseases. Many of the beneficial juices contain vitamins, minerals, and antioxidants which can help to reduce inflammation, boost immunity, and improve kidney health.

Cranberry juice is one of the most popular juices for managing kidney diseases. It contains compounds called proantho-cyanidins which can help to prevent bacteria from sticking to the walls of the urinary tract, reducing the risk of infections.

Prune juice is also beneficial for kidney health as it is high in antioxidants and can help to reduce inflammation.

Other juices such as beet, pomegranate, apple, and grape juice can also help to improve kidney health. These juices are rich in vitamins and minerals which can help to support kidney function and reduce the risk of further damage.

Cranberry juice

Ingredients:

• 1 cup fresh cranberries

• 1 cup of water

• 2 tablespoons of honey

• 1/4 teaspoon of ground ginger

Instructions:

1. Rinse the cranberries and place them in a medium-sized pot.

2. Add the water and bring to a boil over medium-high heat.

3. Reduce the heat to low and simmer for 10 minutes.

4. Strain the mixture through a fine-mesh sieve to remove the cranberry skins and seeds.

5. Add the honey and ground ginger to the cranberry juice and stir to combine.

6. Serve chilled or over ice. Enjoy!

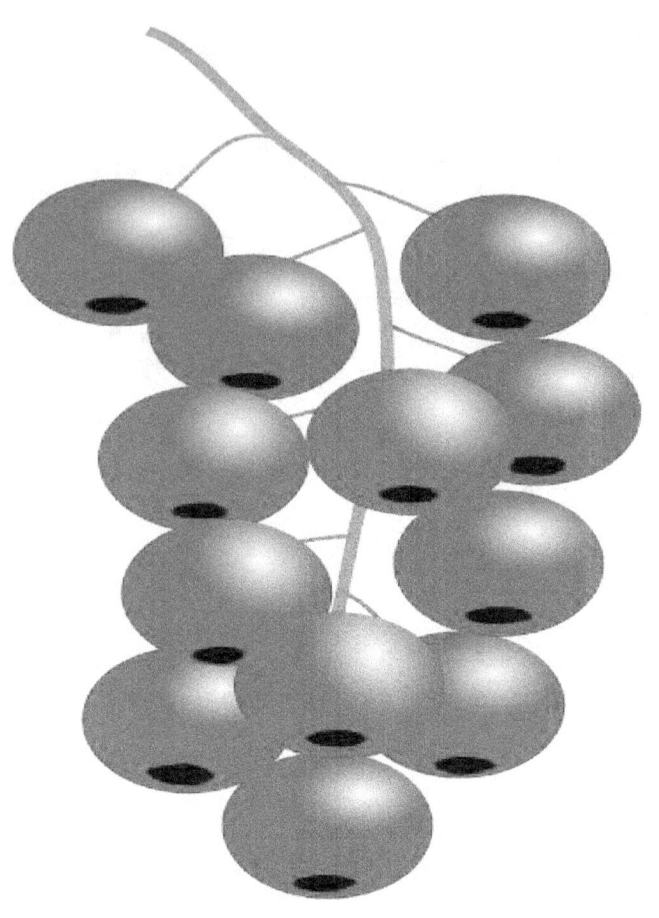

Benefits of cranberry juice for kidney health

Cranberry juice contains high levels of vitamin C and other antioxidants, which can help protect your kidneys from oxidative damage. The juice also contains compounds known as proanthocyanidins, which have been found to reduce the risk of urinary tract infections. This is important because infections in the urinary tract can spread to the kidneys and cause damage.

Prune juice

Ingredients:

- 2 pounds of pitted prunes

- 4 cups of water

- 1/4 cup of honey

- Juice of 1 lemon

Instructions:

1. Place the prunes in a medium-sized saucepan.

2. Pour the water over the prunes and bring to a boil over medium-high heat.

3. Reduce the heat to low and simmer for 30 minutes, stirring occasionally.

4. Remove the pan from the heat and allow the mixture to cool.

5. Place the prunes and liquid into a blender and blend until smooth.

6. Strain the mixture through a fine-mesh sieve into a pitcher.

7. Add the honey and lemon juice to the pitcher and stir until combined.

8. Pour the prune juice into glasses and serve chilled. Enjoy!

Prune juice health benefit for kidney health

Prune juice has long been associated with promoting good kidney health. This is due to its high content of vitamins and minerals, as well as its natural diuretic properties.

Studies have shown that prune juice can help reduce the risk of kidney stones and urinary tract infections.

It is also believed to help lower blood pressure and reduce the risk of developing kidney disease. Prune juice is rich in potassium, which is important for maintaining healthy kidney function. Potassium helps the kidneys to flush out toxins and waste products from the body.

It helps to maintain the body's electrolyte balance, which is important for optimal kidney function. In addition, prune juice is a good source of soluble fiber, which helps to keep the kidneys functioning properly.

Fiber helps to reduce the amount of cholesterol in the body, which can help reduce the risk of kidney stones. Finally, prune juice is a natural diuretic, which helps to increase the rate at which fluids are filtered through the kidneys. This helps to flush out excess toxins and waste products, improving overall kidney health.

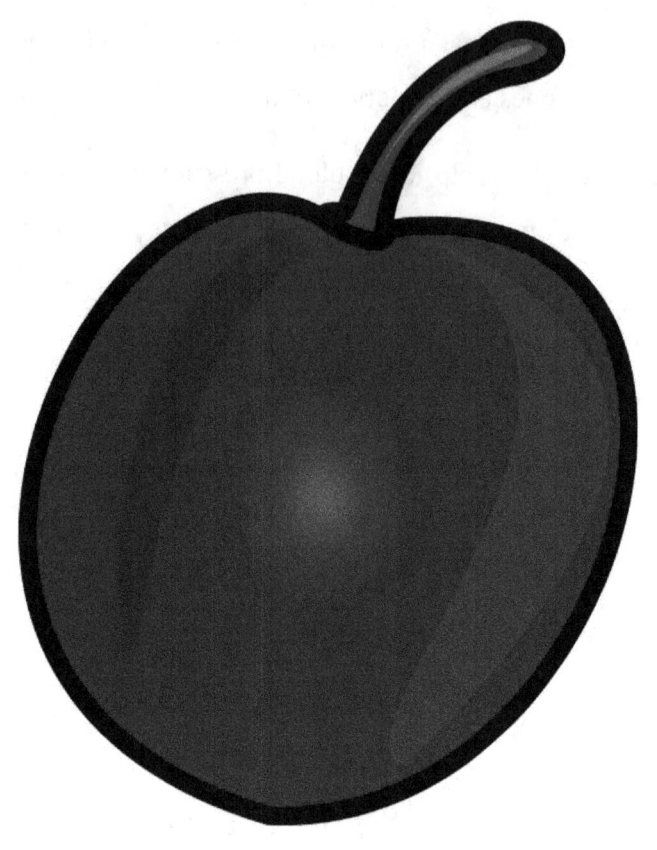

Apple Juice

Ingredients:

- 4 large organic apples

- 1 tablespoon of organic lemon juice

- 2 tablespoons of organic honey

- 2 cups of purified water

- 2 cinnamon sticks

Instructions

1. Wash the apples and cut each one into eight slices.

2. Place the slices in a blender, along with the lemon juice, honey and water.

3. Blend until smooth.

4. Pour the apple juice into a large pot.

5. Add the cinnamon sticks and bring to a boil.

6. Reduce the heat and simmer for 10 minutes.

7. Strain the juice into a pitcher and discard the cinnamon sticks.

8. Serve warm or chilled and enjoy!

Benefits of Apple Juice for kidney Health

Apple juice is rich in potassium, which helps to maintain the electrolyte balance in the body. It also helps to flush out toxins and reduce inflammation. The lemon juice helps to alkalize the body and the honey is a natural sweetener that helps to boost the immune system. The cinnamon sticks add a warm, spicy flavour to the drink and provide ant-inflammatory and antioxidant benefits.

Beet Juice

Ingredients:

- 2 medium beets, peeled and chopped

- 2 carrots, peeled and chopped

- 2 stalks of celery, chopped

- 2 cups of water

- 1/2 cup of freshly squeezed lemon juice

- 1/4 teaspoon of sea salt

Instructions:

1. Place all ingredients into a blender and blend until smooth.

2. Strain the mixture into a glass.

3. Drink the juice immediately or store in the refrigerator in an airtight container for up to 2-3 days.

4. Enjoy!

Benefits of Beet Juice for Kidney Health

Beet juice is a great way to support kidney health. It contains antioxidants, anti-inflammatory compounds, and minerals that can help to cleanse the kidneys and flush out toxins. Additionally, beets are high in dietary nitrates, which can help to reduce inflammation, improve blood flow to the kidneys, and improve kidney function.

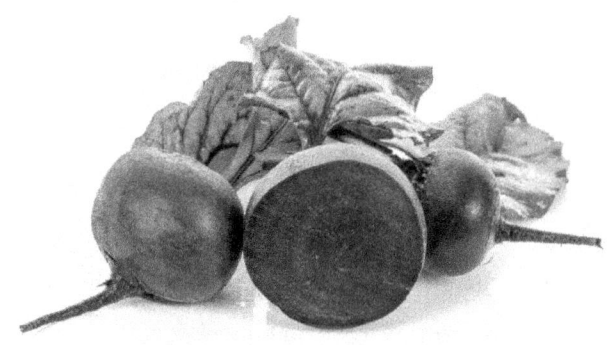

Grape Juice

Ingredients:

• 6 cups of fresh, seedless grapes

• 2 cups of water

• 1/2 cup of honey, or to taste

• 1/2 cup of lemon juice

• 1 teaspoon of ground cinnamon

• 1/2 teaspoon of ground ginger

• Pinch of nutmeg

• Ice cubes (optional)

Instructions:

1. Wash the grapes and remove any stems and leaves.

2. Put the grapes in a blender and blend until smooth.

3. Add the water, honey, lemon juice, cinnamon, ginger, and nutmeg and blend for a few seconds until combined.

4. Strain the juice through a fine-mesh sieve or cheesecloth to remove any solids.

5. Pour the juice into glasses and add ice cubes, if desired.

6. Enjoy!

Benefits of Grape Juice for Kidney Health

Grape juice is high in antioxidants and polyphenols, which help protect against damage to the kidneys and other organs.

It also contains potassium and magnesium, which help to maintain healthy blood pressure levels. Also, grape juice is an excellent source of vitamin C, which helps to reduce inflammation and support the immune system.

Greens (vegetables) Juice

Ingredients:

- 1 cup kale

- 1 cup spinach

- ½ cup cucumber

- ½ cup celery

- ½ cup parsley

- 1 cup of water

- 1 lemon

Instructions:

1. Wash and prepare all ingredients.

2. Juice all the ingredients, except for the lemon, in a juicer or blender.

3. Squeeze the lemon juice into the mixture.

4. Serve the juice cold or warm. Enjoy!

Benefis of vegetable juice for kidney health

This recipe is packed with important vitamins, minerals, and antioxidants that are essential for kidney health. Kale and spinach are high in vitamin K, which helps the body to process calcium. Cucumber and celery contain potassium, which helps to maintain healthy kidneys. Parsley is high in vitamin C and helps to flush toxins from the body. Drinking this delicious green juice regularly will help to keep your kidneys healthy and in top shape!

Pomegranate juice

Ingredients:

-1 pomegranate, seeded

-1 cup freshly squeezed orange juice

-1/2 cup freshly squeezed lemon juice

-1/4 cup honey

-1/4 cup water

-1/4 cup ice

Instructions:

1. Begin by seeding the pomegranate. Cut the pomegranate in half, and then hold one half in your hand over a bowl. Tap the pomegranate with a spoon until the seeds fall into the bowl.

2. In a blender, combine the pomegranate seeds, orange juice, lemon juice, honey, and water. Blend until all of the ingredients are thoroughly combined.

3. Pour the juice into a glass, and then add the ice. Stir the juice to combine, and then enjoy!

Pomegranate juice for kidney health

This pomegranate juice recipe is a delicious and nutritious way to support your kidney health. The powerful antioxidants found in the pomegranate are key to helping protect the kidneys from oxidative damage and inflammation. Enjoy this juice as part of a healthy and balanced diet to help keep your kidneys healthy and functioning optimally.

CONCLUSION

Chronic kidney disease (CKD) is a long-term, progressive disease that affects the kidneys, causing them to lose their ability to filter waste and toxins from the body.

It can lead to severe health problems, including anemia, high blood pressure, bone disease, and heart disease. While there is no cure, there are ways to manage CKD and help slow its progression.

One of these is to include natural fruit juices in your diet. Fruit juices are high in antioxidants and other nutrients that can help protect and strengthen your kidneys.

They are also a great source of hydration, which is important for those with CKD. Cranberry juice, for example, has been shown to reduce the risk of urinary tract infections, which can worsen CKD.

Other juices, such as grape and pomegranate juice, may also help slow the progression of kidney disease. In addition to their health benefits, natural fruit juices are also low in sodium, fat, and calories, making them a great choice for those with CKD. You can also mix them with water to create a refreshing and hydrating drink.

When it comes to managing CKD, natural fruit juices can be a great addition to your diet. They are a good source of essential nutrients and can help protect your kidneys from further damage.

However, it is important to speak to your doctor before making any drastic changes to your diet. They can help you create an individualized plan that is tailored to your specific needs and lifestyle.

www.ingramcontent.com/pod-product-compliance
Lightning Source LLC
Chambersburg PA
CBHW070521220526
45467CB00002B/780